8 Effective Yoga Postures to Lose Belly Fat

With pictures of each pose

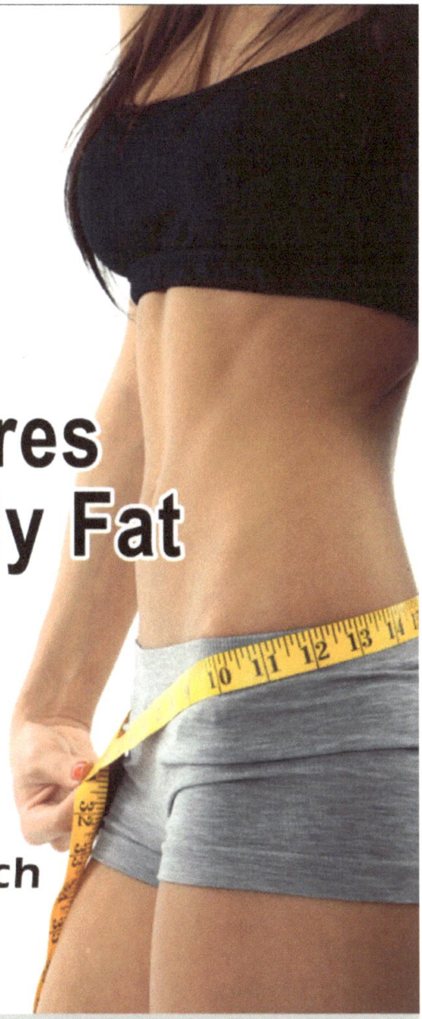

A healthy way of getting a flat stomach at home without spending a penny!

Suchi Gupta

8 Effective Yoga Postures

to

Lose Belly Fat!

By Suchi Gupta

8 Effective Yoga Postures to Lose Belly Fat!

Dedicated to YOU!

May you achieve your goal of having a flat stomach very soon!

That's my wish for you!

Table Of Contents

Acknowledgements

I wish to thank my husband Saket for always showing confidence in me. That matters a lot to me.

A big thank you to my families for giving me time and support always. It really helped me while I was busy creating this book.

A very special thanks to Dr. Ken Evoy and everyone at Site Build It! for sharing their expertise and giving advice and guidance on creating this book and in building my site.

I thank the universe every day for all the wonderful people, things and events in my life.

I wish you the best on your journey to a perfectly flat tummy!

A healthy way of getting flat stomach at home without spending a penny!

Plus a bonus Yoga posture to keep the whole body healthy and flexible always!

Introduction

No need to go to the **gym**.

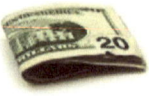

No need to spend your hard earned **money**   to burn stomach fat.

Just try these Yoga postures **at home** and get flat abs in a healthy way!

No-hype at all!

And to make it easy, I have shown **pictures** of each Yoga posture so that you know exactly how it needs to be done. That will also make for an interesting read.

Plus I have sprinkled some practical **tips** to help you maintain a flat tummy always.

And…

…some **tricks** to keep you motivated in your journey to lose stomach fat!

The most **effective** postures are listed first – the ones that worked best for me!

Check out which ones work best for you!

How to get the most out of this book

--Perform the poses when you go through this book. Do not just read the book and see the pictures. **Take action**!

--Do these postures as many number of times as you can. I have written 5-7 or 10-15 depending on the posture. But as time passes you need to increase the repetitions.

--For some days do these "aasanas". Then decide which ones works best for you, not the easiest ones but the most effective ones :)

--**Continue** doing the poses even when you get flat stomach that you always wanted. Do not stop doing them else you will start seeing that fat belly appear again in no time.

--Keep the book handy so that you can go back to it if you need to.

Before you start, Take care!

--**Breathing** is very important for Yoga to be effective, for that matter any exercise to be effective.

We sometimes forget to breathe or stop breathing for a while when we exercise (I do that too) but we must remember to breathe! It's important.

--We tend to over-do Yoga thinking we will get the results faster, but that only hurts the body.

Everybody's body has different limits. Give your body time. Listen to it! **Do not rush. Do not overdo** these poses.

Do them just right so that you feel your abs stretching, but not to a point where it's discomforting.

--Everybody's body type is different. Nobody can promise a **time frame** in which your belly will become flat. Perseverance rules!

--Eat what you love…

… but in moderation, not in excess so that you are not craving for what you love to eat and at the same time have a flat belly! Balance is the key here.

--Losing just stomach fat should not be your aim. The complete body needs to be toned. So, that should really be your goal.

--It's not necessary to do all of these Yoga postures. You can choose the ones that work for you. Postures 1 and 2 did wonders for me!

--If you feel **pain**, please discontinue doing these postures and consult your doctor before starting them again.

--If you are expecting a baby or have some **illness**, please do not try these postures. Consult your doctor/Yoga instructor first.

--These postures are specifically to burn belly fat, they are not " How to lose weight fast " techniques.

Ok, that's enough word of caution. So, are you ready? Great! Lets' start with...

The 8 Yoga Postures to Lose Belly Fat

Lift Your Legs

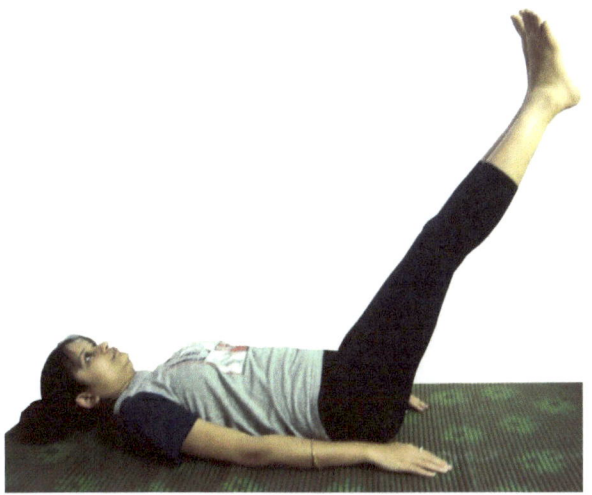

How To Do:

--Lie down on your back and place your arms by your side.

--Now breathe in and lift your legs up in the air, as much as you can. Ideally they should be straight up in the air perpendicular to the rest of your body.

--Breathe out slowly while lowering your legs, but do not touch them on the floor/mat just keep them a little above, in the air.

--Now again breathe in, lift your legs up and repeat.

--Do this for 10-15 times in one go.

--Relax for a few seconds after that.

--Repeat this posture again 5-7 times.

This posture is also known as "Chalit Uttan Padasana". I found this posture very effective in loosing stomach fat!

Ok, now it's time for a quick flat stomach tip. Here we go...

In your daily life, sit with your back straight –Don't droop. That helps in keeping the tummy flat

Toe Crunch

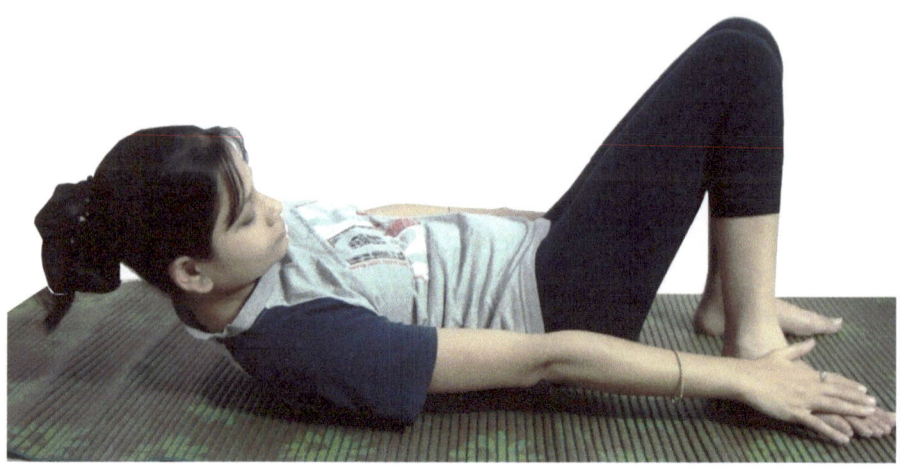

How To Do:

--Lie down on your back and place your arms by your side.

--Now bend your legs bringing your feet towards your hips.

--Lift your shoulders and touch your right feet's thumb with your right hand as shown in the picture above.

--Then touch your left feet's thumb with your left hand.

--Make sure you do not rest your head on the floor/mat in between touching the feet.

--Repeat this for 20-25 times.

--Relax for a few seconds. Repeat this posture for 5-7 times again.

--Keep breathing while doing this.

This is another one which really helped me burn stomach fat fast.

You will actually be able to feel your stomach churn when you do this one. Try it out!

Cross Legs Posture

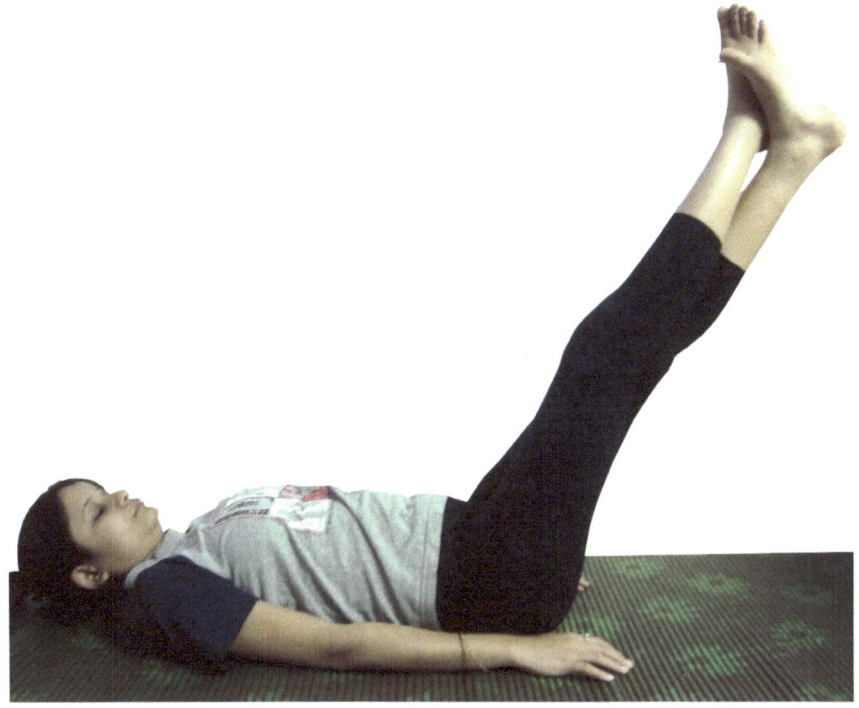

How To Do:

--Lie down on your back and place your arms by your side.

--Now life your legs up in the air, not perpendicular to the rest of your body, just half way.

--Now lift one of the legs a little higher and keep it on top of the other leg as in the picture above.

--Maintain this pose for as long as you can.

--Return to the starting position and relax for a few seconds.

--Repeat this posture for the other leg.

--Relax for a few seconds.

--Repeat this posture 5-7 times for both legs.

--Keep breathing while doing this posture

Another tip on how to lose belly fat and to make these postures more effective…

While doing these Yoga postures, FOCUS on your tummy.

That's the key!

Full Body Stretch

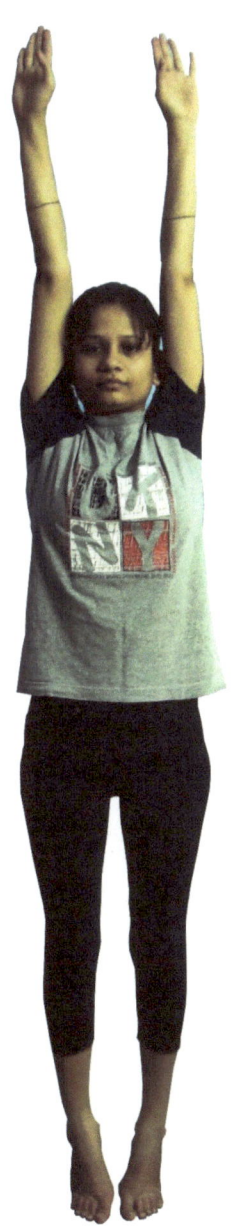

How To Do:

--Stand straight.

--Now breathe in while lifting your hands up and standing on your toes. Not feet, but toes.

--Stretch up as high as you comfortably can like in the picture above.

--Hold your breath for a few seconds while keeping your body stretched.

--Feel your abs stretching.

--Gently exhale as you slowly bring yourself to the starting position.

--Relax for a few seconds. Repeat this posture for 10-15 times again.

This posture is known as "Taad-aasana". "Taad" means tree in Hindi language!

Toe Circles

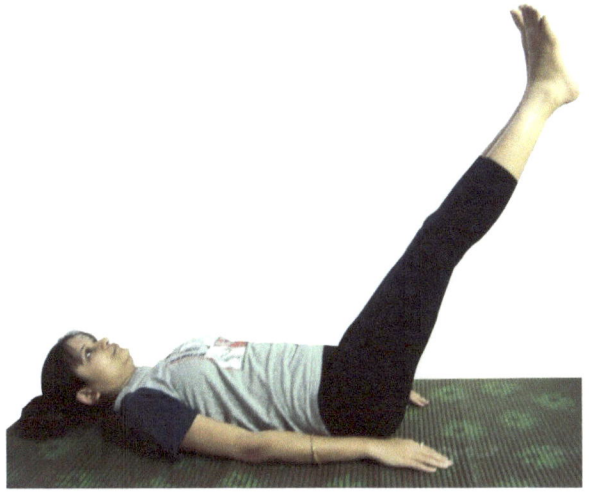

How To Do:

--Lie down on your back and place your arms by your side.

--Now lift your legs up in the air, not straight up, just half way like in the picture above.

--Now keep your legs together and move them clockwise or anti clockwise, as if you are making little circles in the air.

--Repeat this for 10-15 circles.

--Relax for a few seconds. Repeat this posture for 5-7 times again.

--Keep breathing while doing this.

Did you know…

Too much water after meals results in stomach bloating. So, just take a sip or two, not a tumbler full.

The Reverse Boat Pose

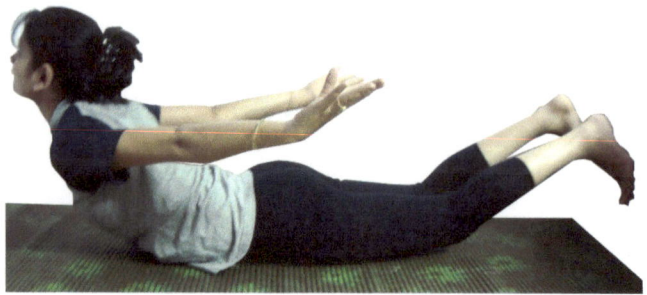

How To Do:

--Lie down with your chin on the floor.

--Inhale and stretch your arms and legs so that your abdomen is the only part of your body that is touching the floor as in the picture above.

--Stay in that position for as long as you can. Keep breathing.

--Exhale and return to the starting position

--Relax for a few seconds and repeat.

This posture is known as "Vipreet Nauka-aasana"

You will feel the pressure on your stomach while you breathe in this pose.

The Bow Pose

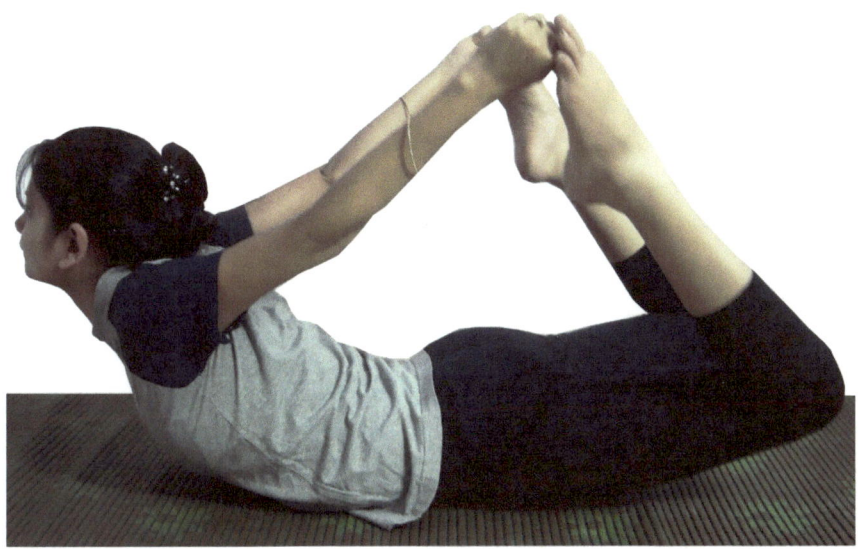

How To Do:

--Lie on your stomach with your chin on the floor.

--Lift your legs up.

--Reach to your feet's thumbs with your arms and grab the right thumb with the right hand and the left thumb with the left hand.

--Slowly inhale and raise your legs by pulling the ankles up and lifting the knees off the floor while raising your chest off the floor at the same time as in the picture above.

--The weight of your body should rest on the stomach completely.

--Tilt your head as far back as possible.

--Slowly exhale and release the thumbs, bring the legs and arms straight down on the floor.

--Relax for a few seconds and repeat.

You may grab your ankles instead of your thumbs.

This posture is known as "Dhanur-aasana".

This one stretches the whole body.

Cobra Pose

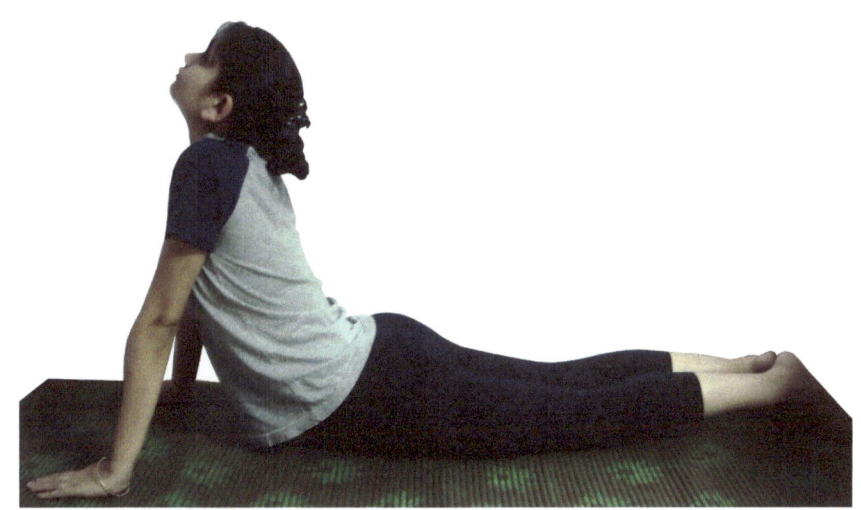

How To Do:

--Lie on the stomach with your chin on the floor and place your arms by your side.

--Bend your arms, inhale and lift your shoulders and head while keeping your torso on the floor as shown in the picture.

--Stretch your head as far back as possible.

--Hold the posture for as long as you can.

--Exhale and return to the starting position slowly.

--Relax for a few seconds and repeat.

This posture is known as "Bhujang-aasana"

How much time will it take every day?

Time Matters…especially in the morning, I know!

Ok…so, let's say you found 4 of these postures effective for yourself…Now let's look at how much time it will take every day to do these...

Posture	Step	Time taken for this step (in seconds)	Total time for the posture (in seconds)
Lift your legs	Lie down with your legs straight	2	2
	Lift your legs up and then down– 1 time	1.5	1.5
	Number of times in one go	15	1.5*15
	Relax	5	1.5*15+5
	No. of Rounds of above steps	3	2+3*((1.5*15)+5)= 84.5
Toes Crunch	Lie down and bend your legs	2	2
	Touch right and then left thumb of your feet	2	2
	No. of times	15	2+2*15=32

Cross your legs	Lie down with your legs straight	2	2
	Lift your legs and cross them	2	2
	Maintain the pose	10	2+10
	Relax	5	2+10+5
	No. of times	5	2 + 5*(2+ 10+5) = 87
Bow pose	Coming into the bow pose	3	3
	Maintain the pose	10	3+10
	Relax	5	3 + 10 + 5
	No. of times	5	5* (3 + 10 + 5) = 90

Now let's take 5 seconds of relaxation time in between these postures, the total time

 comes out to be…

84.5 + 5 + 32 + 5 + 87 + 5 + 90 + 5 = 313.5 seconds, which is about 5.5 minutes.

So, it will take about 6 minutes of your time every morning to achieve your goal of a perfectly flat stomach! Yay!!! :)

Do keep in mind that this is what it takes me to do these postures. The time may vary depending on how flexible one's body is and on the postures you find effective for yourself. Plus you must increase repetitions as time goes by.

Important Tips to Flatten Your Stomach

The Mind Games

Visualization

This works wonders and will keep you motivated!

"You have the perfect figure you always dreamt of."

"You look great in that sexy dress."

"People take tips from you about what you do to maintain that hourglass figure."

Now close your eyes

  …and just imagine these things..

Would you love to get your navel pierced? Well, go ahead and imagine that too!

Wow! That feels great…Isn't it?

Now, let's observe what our thoughts are when we wake up in the morning and think about exercising…

"I want more sleep."

"Aww…I will start from tomorrow, I promise. Not today , pleeaase"

True?

This happens with almost all of us. Now what we can do here is…

At the moment when you wake up, just imagine the above things, think of the compliments, praises and people asking you for tips. You are sure to feel motivated to get up right and continue your journey to that PERFECTLY FLAT STOMACH!!!

That will give your will-power some exercise too! :)

And here are …

Some more tips for motivation!

You can do so many things to keep yourself motivated.

--Get yourself that lovely sexy dress. Don't feel like buying it because you will not be able to wear it? How about making it your aim to wear it to a party looking gorgeous in it? Promise that to yourself and go ahead with these effective yoga postures. Imagine yourself in that wonderful dress.

--Imagine the compliments your loved ones will pour you with…

--Get a picture of your ideal-figure person and place it somewhere so that you can see it every now and then and feel inspired.

--Set up a goal

…with a date - to get your stomach flat. Goal setting is important.

--Imagine how stunning you will look in all the dresses you love to wear…

--Imagine people taking tips from you on "Wow!!! You look great! How did you do it?"

--Feel the feeling of achievement that you will have after you've done it!

…and so on…add to the list whatever works for you…

Plus it will help a lot to…

Think Flat Stomach

Thoughts like…

"I have to lose weight"

"I don't look good"

"I look fat"… will not do any good.

By thinking such thoughts, you are concentrating on weight and you notice "I do not look good."

Now let's try this…just close your eyes, imagine you have that perfect belly already, you are standing in front of a full length mirror looking at yourself. Now, really feel these feelings…

"Wow! I look gorgeous!"

"I have the perfect weight"

"I have a wonderful sexy hourglass figure"

Felt any better?

Such positive thoughts make us feel good about ourselves and take away the focus from weight and bulging tummy. That helps in reducing the fat around the tummy and the result..? A perfect sexy flat stomach!!!

Try it! Close your eyes and feel happy about yourself!

In essence, you need to **make believe** that you have that flat tummy already!

"Feel In-shape".

"Surya Namaskaar"
The Master Yoga Posture

Surya Namaskaar is a series of 12 postures to be done one after the other.

The postures are as shown in the below picture. Completing all 12 postures makes one cycle.

This cycle can be done 2-3 times in the starting, increasing it slowly as the body becomes more flexible.

This series of postures is very helpful for the complete body.

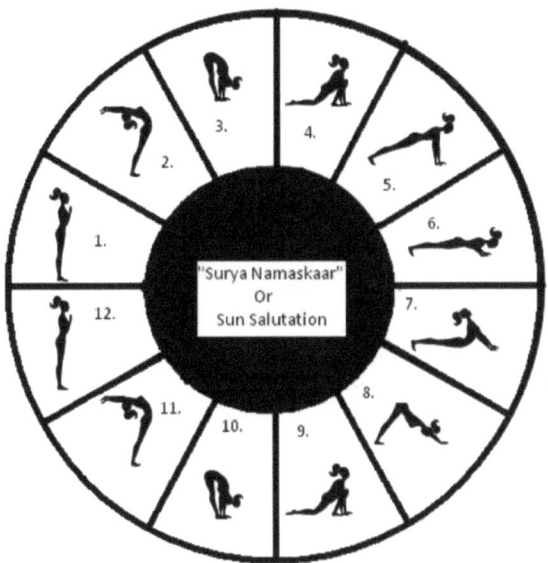

In the starting you will have to remember the sequence of postures but after sometime it will become a habit!

Here are just some..

Benefits of Surya Namaskaar

--It helps reduce feeling of restlessness and **anxiety**, stress and tension.

--Improves **concentration**.

--Helps those who suffer from insomnia or have **disturbed sleep**.

--Regular practice of Surya Namaskaar is the **natural** and easiest way to be in shape. It makes the body flexible, especially the Spinal cord.

--Helps to lose excessive belly fat and gives flat stomach.

--Boosts blood circulation. It is a natural solution to prevent onset of wrinkles and also adds **glow to the face**.

--It is **relaxing** and rejuvenating.

--It helps in improving **digestion**.

--It is helpful in improving the functioning of thyroid, parathyroid and pituitary glands.

--It is good for the **respiratory** system.

--It boosts **endurance** power and...

--Regulates **irregular menstrual cycles**.

--It ensures easy **childbirth**. It helps to decrease the fear of pregnancy and childbirth.

--Helps preventing **hair graying**, hair fall, and dandruff.

--Improves the growth of hair.

Why do Yoga – The Benefits

You would say flat belly! :) Of course, but that's just one of the many benefits.

Along with that, there are a lot of benefits you will get if you do these Yoga poses regularly.

Here are some…

--The excess fat around the thighs and buttocks will disappear, giving you **a sexy figure.**

--Your **spine** will be strengthened. Spine is a VERY important part of our body, rightly called the "Backbone". These postures will strengthen your backbone.

--Feel **fresh** as these "aasanas" (postures are called "aasanas" in Hindi language) provide relief in constipation problems too because the pressure is applied on the stomach.

--**Gas** troubles are also resolved if these "aasanas" are done on a regular basis.

--You would have **glowing skin** as these "aasanas" increase circulation of blood to the entire body.

--These postures also improve **respiratory** problems.

--Have a job with very little movement? Like sitting in front of the computer for a long time…? Try these "aasanas" and you would be relieved from **stiffness** in shoulders. Plus frozen shoulder conditions are also improved.

--Feel light as Yoga improves **digestion** too!

--Yoga strengthens **concentration** and mental **determination**. That will help you achieve more in lesser time!

--It helps develop internal **balance and harmony**.

--Yoga improves functioning of **kidneys and liver**, increasing your life!!!

About the Author

Hi there!

I'm Suchi from India. I have had a thin body always except flab on my stomach. That looked bad!

I went all over the internet looking for exercises to reduce the belly fat. Everywhere I found there was a description of what needs to be done without any images showing what exactly needs to be done. Many times I was not even able to understand what I'm supposed to do.

So, I made sure I have pictures for each posture so you do not have to face the problem that I faced.

I wanted a flat stomach in a healthy way, no dieting or saying to 'No' to foods I love to eat...plus something that I could do at home...without spending my money. Yoga was the solution to all these!

I have benefitted from these Yoga postures and got rid of my belly fat. So, I thought why not share my experiences with the world out there so everybody including you can benefit from these.

And since keeping myself motivated to get out of bed and do these postures was the most difficult part for me, I have added here the tricks that worked for me.

So, here's the book for you - a compilation of healthy flat stomach exercises which can be done at home without the need to spend money.

I truly hope you also find it helpful in losing stomach fat. Anyone can do it...just a little bit of PATIENCE is required!

Would you like to share your flat-tummy-experiences with me? Please drop a line at replytosuchi [at] yahoo dot com. I would love to hear from you!

All the very best for your journey towards a flat and sexy stomach! :)

Suchi Gupta

Attributions

The pictures that I have used in this "how to burn belly fat" book have been taken from http://www.sxc.hu. They have been clicked by:

Foxumon - The money picture

Nadia Jasmine – The cake picture

Sandy Yin – The eyes closed picture

Jaylopez – The Goal picture

Tom Pickering - The patience picture

Ivan Prole – The time picture

Thanks to all these wonderful photographers!